Health Healing Food and Herbal Medicine:

Health Healing or Disease and Physical Ailment

ERNIE ONG

Text Copyright © ERNIE ONG

Legal & Disclaimer

The information in this book and its contents is not designed to replace nor take the place of any form of medical or professional advice; it is not meant to replace the need for independent medical, financial, legal, or other professional advice or services, as may be required. The content and information in this book have been provided for educational and entertainment purposes only.

The content and information in this book have been compiled from sources deemed reliable, and they are accurate to the best of the author's knowledge, information, and beliefs. However, the author cannot guarantee its accuracy and validity and cannot be held liable for any errors and/or omissions. Furthermore, changes are periodically made to this book as and when needed. Where appropriate and/or necessary, you must consult a professional (including but not limited to your doctor, attorney, financial advisor, or other professional advisors) before using any of the suggested remedies, techniques, or information in this book.

Upon using the contents and information in this book, you agree to hold harmless the author from and against any damages, costs, and expenses, including any legal fees potentially resulting from the application of any of the information provided by this book. This disclaimer applies to any loss, damages, or injury caused by the use and application, whether directly or indirectly, of any advice or information presented, whether for breach of contract, tort, negligence, personal injury, criminal intent, or under any other cause of action.
You agree to accept all risks of using the information presented inside this book.

You agree that by continuing to read this book, where appropriate and/or necessary, you shall consult a professional (including but not limited to your doctor, attorney, or financial advisor or other advisors as needed) before using any of the suggested remedies, techniques, or information in this book. While the book refers to real-life situations, the names mentioned may have been changed.

Table of Contents

Introduction

Welcome to the University of Life. We have lots of fun and entertainment for everyone to learn archery, shoot paintballs, war games, hunting, fishing, lots, and lots of trees to be chopped down, and the Ecosystem will continue to be destroyed. The Economy comes first.

We will kill all the animals in the forest, all the fishes in the ocean, ignoring global warming.

Arctic ice, trapping viruses for millions of years, is melting, and the sea level is rising. Humans are kings over the mountains, oceans, and all living creatures on earth. We are hunters everywhere with drought on the farmlands and floods in the cities. With everything almost gone - humans start harming humans. Humans are beings with an inhuman nature.

Mother Nature is fighting back, releasing a virus that will kill millions. Humans start collecting these viruses to keep and profit from them to solve their political, economic, military, and social population problems; terrorism is another problem. The worse is yet to come. Every problem is only the beginning.

Time is on the side of change. The hunters will now become the hunted. The virus became a global pandemic, and many people are saying it is only mild flu. The virus is everywhere and will take, especially the old, the poor, and the sick.

This writer is an ex-military trainer of an elite fighting force in Singapore and a taxi driver at this present moment. Having to serve all the front liners and passengers in essential services every day is a mind-blogging affair.

Many people fall sick every day. I hope to depart to you the knowledge of how I keep as safe and healthy as possible, being in the frontline ferrying people for essential services every day.

In the Military, you have to be safe, observant, disciplined, and prepared. You have to use your head, be alert, analyze, optimistic, quick, and decisive.

You are fighting an invisible enemy. Like all soldiers, you will be taught to endure and survive, not get run down by a car, or attempt suicide with detergent. When you are in a fight, even if you could not kill your enemy, you must weaken your enemy.

Strengthen your bodies with exercise, sunlight, oxygen, hydrogen water, alkaline water, micronutrients, metabolites, yoga, Qi, and many other natural remedies.

We will do whatever we can to learn about our enemy and improve our health until the vaccine is ready. Do you want to save yourself? Gain knowledge, read on.

Chapter 1 - The Secret to Longevity

"If you ask what the single most important key to longevity is, I would have to say it is avoiding worry, stress, and tension. And if you didn't ask me, I'd still have to say it." - George Burns

Many people believe that longevity is pegged to our genetic makeup. So what happens when you have weak family genetics? Does it mean you are doomed? The good news is your genetics only contribute a small part to your life expectancy. The best part is there are many other factors you can improve, such as your lifestyle, diet, and habits.

According to The Medical Classic of the Yellow Emperor Journal of Internal Medicine, written by the famous Chinese Haungdi around 2600 BC, the secret of longevity is to follow the Tao, which is the natural way of the universe. Your body is a balance of two fundamental forces known as yin and yang, influenced primarily by five elements known as earth, water, wood, metal, fire, and the organs of your body. Simply put, to maintain balance in your body, get ample sunlight, cool fresh air, clean, freshwater, and adequate sleep followed by proper exercise and meditation.

Sunlight

Did you know that research shows 40 percent of American adults suffer from vitamin D deficiency? Low vitamin D can lead to serious side effects and health consequences, such as infections, immune system disorders, fatigue, depression, osteoporosis, diabetes, cancer, and muscle weakness.

Why you need vitamin D:

- Strengthens the immune system that helps you fight off harmful infections, viruses, and bacteria, such as influenza and Covid-19.

- Strengthens and promote bone growth by enhancing the absorption of calcium in your gut.

- Decreases the risk of weak muscles and falls, which is a common problem for the elderly.

- Supports oral health by decreasing the risk of gum disease and tooth decay.

- Prevents diabetes by helping to lower the risk of an over-abundance of sugar in your blood.

- According to a Neuropsychology journal, vitamin D helps to brighten your mood and improve patients suffering from depression.

- According to the National Cancer Institute (NCI), there is evidence that vitamin D helps lower risks in certain cancers, such as breast, prostate, colorectal, and pancreatic.

Most doctors advise the recommended amount of vitamin D is 1000 to 2000 IU daily. The only way to know if your vitamin D is adequate is to be diagnosed through a simple blood test.

The sun is your best source of vitamin D because the sun's ultraviolet B (UVB) rays help synthesis the production of vitamin D. Research shows that 10 am to 3 pm is the most optimum time for absorbing vitamin D. Depending on which part of the planet you live, around 15 to 30 minutes of midday sun exposure three times weekly is sufficient to maintain healthy levels of vitamin D for most people. For example, if you are fair or pale-skinned, you only need 10 to 15 minutes of sunlight versus a dark-skinned person who might need extended time.

Another alternative to getting enough vitamin D is through foods such as:

- Fatty fish, e.g., tuna, salmon, sardines, and mackerel.

- Fortified vitamin D foods, such as cereals, yogurt, milk, and orange juice.

- Vitamin D supplements containing 800 to 2000 IUs daily.

Fresh Air

One of life's simple pleasures is a breath of fresh air. Science has shown us that getting some fresh outdoor air has benefits such as:

- Improves digestion by supplying your stomach and intestines with blood flow.

- It helps you feel relaxed and happier, thus preventing depression.

- Improves recovery time by helping you heal faster from injuries and illness because your body's damaged cells need fresh oxygen.

- Improves your circulatory systems and overall health.

- Cleanses your lungs and releases toxins from your body.

- It gives you oxygen to help you fight off tiredness and stress.

- Gets more oxygen to your brain, thus giving you a sharper mind to focus on your tasks.

When you feel yourself getting sluggish or off-center, step outside and take a few good deep breaths of fresh air, and your body will thank you for it.

Water

Did you know that your body comprises of 60 percent water, and only 2 percent of dehydration can cause you to feel thirsty and experience dizziness, headaches, and nausea?

Water is one of the most vital nutrients you need because it helps to:

- Regulate your internal body temperature through respiration and sweating.

- Metabolize and transport the carbohydrates and proteins in your body.

- Reduce burdens on your kidney and liver and eliminating waste through urination.

- Moisturize your eyes, nose, and mouth.

- Lubricate your joints.

- Transport nutrients and oxygen to your cells.

The recommended amount of water is 15.5 cups for men and 11.5 cups for women. If you are taking medicines and supplements, drink adequate water.

Although it is important to drink plenty of water, however, over hydration, water toxemia, also known as water poisoning, offsets the electrolytes in the body and can cause fatal disturbance to the brain functions.

<u>Alkaline Water</u>

In Taiwan, Japan, Korea, and certain parts of China, they make tea with spring water or mountain water, which brings out the taste and antioxidant in the tea. This water carries a higher PH content bringing good health to the drinker. The water is also used for cooking, making beer, bathing, and spa.

If you do not have alkaline water, you can make your own by mixing half a teaspoon of baking soda with a glass of water that gives PH 8.3.
After passing motion, immediately shower to keep clean and safe for everyone at home. Then do a sinus rinse and drink alkaline water from Hengshan, a mountainous region in Taiwan, PH 8.8.

Your blood PH will not be affected and will remain a constant PH 7.3. Any excess will pass through your kidneys and waste after cleaning your urinary system. You can repeat after two hours if necessary.

If your eyes start to itch, you could be drinking too much alkaline water. Take a break.

Sleep

According to a study by the American Academy of Sleep Medicine, one in three Americans does not get regular adequate sleep. The recommended sleep is at least 7 hours to maintain optimal health and wellbeing. Otherwise, you might risk developing diabetes, obesity, heart disease, and high blood pressure.

The National Sleep Foundation recommends sleeping between 8 pm to midnight because it follows your body's natural internal sleep cycle of rapid eye movement (REM) and non-rapid eye movement (NREM). When you are sleeping, your body releases growth hormones to help your body grow and repair itself. If you are ill or injured, your immune system will release cytokines, a type of small proteins to help your body fight infection, inflammation, and trauma. Sleeping also gives your sympathetic nervous systems, known as the fight or flight response, a chance to rest. At the same time, your cortisol level, known as the stress hormone, decreases, thus making you feel refreshed upon waking.

If you do not have adequate sleep, your body cannot do any of the above amazing things to help you function at your best every day.

Exercise

World Health Organization (WHO) recommends 150 minutes of physical activity weekly. You can break it down into 30 minutes of moderate physical activity 5 times weekly, e.g., brisk walking or jogging. Benefits of regular physical activity can help you:

- Lower the risk of heart disease, stroke, high blood pressure, diabetes, osteoporosis, depression, and dementia.

- Maintain a healthy weight, body mass, and composition.

- Improve cardio and muscular fitness.

- If you are only starting to exercise, be patient, start slow, and build up gradually. For example, you can start with brisk walking for warm-up or stairs climbing for improving endurance and stamina.

Caution: Do not exercise if you are not feeling well, have enough sleep, or are intoxicated, especially if you are of age. Insufficient sleep can give you high blood pressure and cause difficulty breathing. Alcohol can cause dehydration, thus causing muscle cramps, or a person can pass out during exercise.

Meditation

Meditation is about relaxation, attention, compassion, training awareness, deep breathing, and emptying of the mind. Try doing some form of meditation regularly to help you reduce stress and anxiety in your life.

A survey was done on seniors above the age of seventy, asking if they have any regrets in life. The most common answer is that they regret wasting time worrying about everything, whether big or small because most of their worries never occurred.

If you find yourself worrying, ask yourself 2 questions:

1) Is it worthwhile to worry about this problem?

2) Will the problem be solved by worrying?

If you know that living is suffering, why suffer some more?
Free the thoughts, free the self.

Chapter 2 - Bioavailability

"Our food should be our medicine and our medicine should be our food."
-Hippocrates

Bioavailability refers to the rate and degree at which a drug or substance is being absorbed into your body.

<u>Vitamin C</u>

Vitamin C is one of the most effective and safest nutrients to take as a cold remedy or flu prevention. The nutrient in vitamin C will boost your immune system helping you to fight the common cold. Vitamin C or ascorbic acid is necessary for growth, development, and the repair of body tissues, bone structure, iron absorption, immune function, wound healing, and healthy skin. Furthermore, it is also an antioxidant that helps protect you against damage caused by free radicals, toxic chemicals, and pollutants, e.g., cigarette smoke. Unfortunately, your body does not produce vitamin C, which is why you need to get your vitamin C from vegetables and citrus fruits, such as orange, grapefruit, lemon, and strawberries, or supplements.

According to a report by Harvard Health, more than 11,000 active participants, including army troops, runners, and skiers who took at least 200mg of vitamin C daily were able to reduce their risk of catching a cold by 50 percent. Moreover, taking at least 200mg of vitamin C can help reduce the duration of cold symptoms by 8 percent, which is the equivalent to one day less of illness.

In a nutshell, if you really want to reap the benefits of vitamin C, you need to consume it daily and not only during the cold season or at the start of cold symptoms.

<u>How much vitamin C should you take?</u>

Doctors recommend 90mg per day for men and 75mg per day for women; this is equivalent to approximately five fruits and vegetables daily. Studies have shown that only 10 to 20 percent of people get the recommended amount of vitamin C from foods daily. Therefore, you must consider taking vitamin C supplements at 500mg daily. Excess vitamin C is excreted, so overdose is usually not a concern. The safe upper limit for vitamin C is 2,000mg daily. Consuming more than 2,000mg may result in diarrhea, nausea, and abdominal pain. It is also best to consume vitamin C supplements that are non-acidic and in a buffered form, so it does not irritate your stomach.

Vitamin D and Magnesium

Vitamin D is also known as the "sunshine vitamin" because it is produced in your skin in response to sunlight. The good news is your body naturally produces vitamin D whenever it is exposed to sunlight. Besides sunlight, you can also get vitamin D from certain foods, such as egg yolk, fatty fish, e.g., salmon and fortified milk or supplements (refer to Chapter 1).

Vitamin D's bioavailability depends on magnesium. The enzymes (in the liver and kidneys) that enable vitamin D metabolism – converting it into its active form, calcitriol – can't work without a sufficient amount of magnesium to draw upon.

Magnesium plays a vital role in determining how much vitamin D your body can produce. It has been suggested that people whose magnesium level is high are less likely to have vitamin D deficiency compared to people with low magnesium levels. Thus taking magnesium supplements will help increase the deficient vitamin D level. The recommended amount of magnesium is 300mg for men and 270mg for women. Do note that too much vitamin D can increase calcium levels and cause health complications. For example, when you exceed your recommended dietary allowance of calcium, it can cause your hormones to draw the mineral out of your bones and deposit it in soft tissues, such as arteries. Note: Magnesium, vitamins, and other minerals all work together and rely on each other to be fully effective. Vitamin D supplements help to keep your muscles healthy, but it won't work effectively in strengthening your bones unless the concentrations of boron, magnesium, and zinc, vitamins K and A, are at the correct levels.

Ultimately, it is important that you maintain a balanced diet by eating a wide variety of foods consisting of plenty of vegetables, fruits, fish, and high fiber starchy carbohydrates, such as whole-wheat, brown rice, and potatoes with skins for different nutrients.

Chapter 3 - Prevention

"Prevention is better than cure" - Desiderius Erasmus

There are no vaccines available for the COVID-19 pandemic at the point of writing, which was first identified in Wuhan, China, in December 2019. Since its outbreak, the virus has already claimed more than one million deaths worldwide.

So far, no medication can kill this virus. We are using science, history, technology, electromagnetism, TCM, Long-Wavelength, Short-Wavelength, Infrared Red Heat, UV lights, Ozone Air, Chorine steam to kill, to sterilize, and weaken the virus.

While waiting for the vaccine, our life still goes on, and the best you can do is reduce your risk of getting the virus by:

- Limiting your exposure to the number of people you meet daily.

- Practicing good personal hygiene to prevent the virus from entering your system.

- Paying attention to any surface areas you touch and sanitize your hands regularly. Because of the SARS virus in 2002, people are now aware that surface areas like lift buttons, handrails, and escalators are highly contagious. For example, the keypad on the credit card payment terminal at the Airport pharmacy was tested and contained the most viruses, germs, and bacteria.

- Wear your face mask for protection and practice social distancing whenever possible. Whenever someone coughs or sneezes, they can expel up to 40,000 droplets into the air. If containing the virus, these droplets can last up to 4 hours on copper surfaces, 24 hours on cardboard, and 2 to 3 days on plastic and stainless steel surfaces. Even toilet flushing can produce droplets called aerosols that can last more than one minute in the air. Note: Studies have shown that COVID-19 is transmitted mostly between person-to-person via physical contact and respiratory droplets.

- The likelihood of viruses surviving outdoors is low. Therefore opt for big open areas with fresh air, as ventilation can avert virus infection versus small confined areas.

Note: Watch out for all other diseases such as New Swine Flu (H1N1) and dengue, which is also rising and fast-spreading.

Caring for Our System in the Body

Your skin, lungs, liver, and kidneys can be detoxified through exercising, perspiration, urination, and excretion. The liver performs more than 500 functions in the body. Not to mention our skin, which is our largest organ yet often neglected. It is time to take good care of your body so it can take good care of you.

Suggestions:

- Do a blood test and discuss with your doctor any excess and shortage of nutrients in your body.

- Do exercise movements for all the joints in your body.

- Get out into the sun where vitamin D and fresh air is in abundance.

- Check on yourself and everything at home. For example, are you using pillows made from microfibers? The latest studies by Chinese researchers found that pillows made from microfibers can be reservoirs for coronavirus and a potential source of virus transmission. A virus can stay from several hours to a few days depending on the room temperature.

- It is easier and more hygiene to use and throw away facial tissue and kitchen towels used for cleaning, instead of keeping the soiled towels and washing them.

- The most important preventive measure is to keep yourself very clean.

- Take immediate action to minimize getting infected. For example, use hand sanitizer after you touch the lift buttons.

Apart from measures from the government, be proactive with your protective measures, such as:

- Wear your face mask. Remind people who don't wear a mask or give one to them. They might have forgotten or lost their mask. Wearing a mask will help prevent the spreading virus to others. However, it is only effective if everyone wears them. Everyone can do their part by not spreading the virus because what goes around comes around.

- Practice good personal hygiene by washing your hands regularly. Keeping your hands clean can prevent illness and viruses effectively. It is especially important to wash your hands before eating and refrain from licking your fingers. Don't forget to trim your fingernails short and keep them clean.

- Whenever you sneeze onto your palms, wash your hands with antiseptic soap. You want to prevent spreading any germs or viruses from your hands to your eyes.

- Cover your mouth if you need to cough. Many people remove their masks to cough and end up releasing droplets into the air. Instead, you can cough into tissue paper and discard it into a Ziplock or airtight container.

- Keep a hand sanitizer with you wherever you go. It is very useful when you do not have access to soap and water. It is good to sanitize or wash your hands whenever you come in contact with other people.

- Avoid touching your face. The virus can spread from your hands and enter through your facial skin, eyes, nose, or ears. Wipe your face with antiseptic wipes or soap after you have touched your face.

- Practice social distancing measures. Keep 1m apart from each other whenever possible. Refrain from talking in crowded places like buses, trains, and markets.

- Regularly disinfect your mobile phone, spectacles, money, and everything before and after you use them. Viruses can survive on cool surfaces like phone screens and money for thirty days.

- Ventilate your home and surrounding by opening windows and doors. The air outside is cleaner and fresher than indoors by as much as ten times.

- Avoid hotspots, such as high traffic areas. A person can be re-infected with COVID-19 twice and be even sicker the second time.

- Exercising as little as 10 minutes a day doing aerobics, walking, or cycling can improve your sleep quality. On the other hand, over-exercising can drain your body of energy and nutrients, weakening your immune system and making you more susceptible to illness.

- Get adequate sleep and rest at least 7 hours. Proper sleep and rest will restore your energy, giving you greater energy, boosting your immune system, and helping you operate at peak performance daily.

- Strengthen your immune system. A strong immune system will help you ward off colds and flu by defending you against any disease-causing micro-organisms. Even if you fall sick, you will experience milder symptoms and recover faster.

- Keep yourself informed by reading books on food nutrition, exercises, health, illness, natural remedies, etc.

- Seek professional medical diagnosis if necessary. For example, whatever I am suggesting in this book may work for me but not for you. For instance, I have sufficient vitamin D, potassium, and magnesium in my body, even though I am considered old. You may be deficient even though you are considered a young man. I am not allergic to anything. Some people are allergic to nuts, seafood, grass, hay, flowers, pollen, etc. Moreover, people who have diabetes, high blood pressure, hypertension, and high cholesterol can be more problematic.

- Some countries implemented movement control orders during this COVID-19 pandemic. People were unable to go to work or stock up on daily essentials. Furthermore, confusion arises when people started hoarding and emptying the supermarkets. Little do they know that the lockdown means food and agriculture workers are not working on farms. For example, some farmers could not get the hay across borders to feed their cattle and sheep, resulting in thousands of farm animals facing starvation. These issues could pose a threat to our global food supply chain. Some countries like Kazakhstan, Vietnam, Serbia, and Romania have temporarily ban food exports of their grains, rice, sunflower oil, and flour. Perhaps this could be prevented if world leaders coordinated a global plan to prepare everyone for the lockdown.

- During COVID-19, avoid going to the hospital unnecessarily because you could be exposing yourself to the virus. Prepare a first aid kit at home so that you do not need to rush to the clinic or hospital unnecessarily.

- During a pandemic, minimize going out. Arrange for non-contact deliveries, have your necessities delivered and left at your door, pick them up after the delivery person has left. Movement control order means you cannot get others to buy things for you if it is a complete lockdown. Supermarkets will be hoarded, and there will be no delivery from restaurants. Be prepared for a total shutdown.

My Immediate Action Plan

Mask up, arrive, and leave as soon as possible. Take with anti-inflammatory and antibacterial lozenges like Difflam to prevent inflammation. Wash your face and clean up in the nearest washroom (I carry two 2L bottles of water in my car as standby).

Put a Fluimucil tablet in water to drink; it will help to reduce mucus. You can also take 2 Uniflu tablets to combat any symptoms associated with cold and flu. These medicines do not require a doctor's prescription but be careful not to overdose (four to six hours between each dosage).

Chapter 4 - Symptoms and Treatments

"Health is not valued till sickness comes." -Thomas Fuller

<u>Detoxification</u>

Detoxification is one of the fastest ways to reduce infection of your cells. The fewer viruses in your body, the fewer symptoms you have to treat. Some patients suffer from multiple organ damages, and a few hundred different symptoms.

The good news is your body system naturally cleanses and detoxes 24 hours a day. Any toxins are naturally excreted through perspiration, urine, stools, and exhalation. To help your body detox better, you can:

- Drink more water.

- Get adequate sleep.

- Avoid alcohol.

- Reduce intake of processed foods, sugar, and salt.

- Eat more antioxidant-rich foods like vitamin C, berries, and nuts.

- Eat more prebiotics high foods like bananas, tomatoes, oats, and artichokes.

- Get active daily; exercise helps you flush out your lungs, increases blood circulation, and cleanses your skin through sweating.

- In China, Traditional Chinese Medicine (TCM) uses Qing Fei Pai Du Tang, a classic traditional Chinese herbal formula to clear the lungs and remove toxins to detox. According to a report by Beijing Traditional Chinese Medicine Hospital, after analyzing 9,600 cases of COVID-19, they prevented mild cases from worsening by using TCM.

- Look out for "dirty dozen" foods that are toxic because of their exposure to pesticides and herbicides. The most common ones are apples, peaches, blueberries, celery, bell peppers, grapes, spinach, lettuce, mushrooms, and potatoes. If you like to eat these foods, opt for organic, wash them, or peel the skin before eating.

- Try eating more carotenoids-rich foods because they contain beneficial antioxidants that boost your immune system and protect you from disease. For example, carrots, tomatoes, yams, kale, papaya, pumpkin, oranges, and mangoes.

- Drug toxicity means there are too many drugs in a person's system; this happens when a person over-ingests or has an adverse drug reaction to medicine. Symptoms can include dizziness, diarrhea, nausea, vomiting, seizures, and slurred speech. Therefore, be careful with any supplements or medicines you are taking and read the labels carefully.

Food Poisoning - Activated Charcoal

Activated charcoal is made from coconut shells, peat, bone char, coal, olive pits, and petroleum coke and processed at high temperatures. It can be used for treating emergency food poisoning or drug overdose. It works by trapping the toxins and chemicals in your gut, preventing their absorption. Since your body cannot absorb activated charcoal, the toxins will be carried out of your body through excretion.

Throat Pain or Throat Infection

- Add half a teaspoon of salt, a tablespoon of sugar in a glass of warm water and stir before drinking.

- Spray Watermelon Frost Powder spray into your mouth where the ulcer resides. You can check where the ulcer is by using a torchlight (you can use your phone) and shine into your mouth while facing the mirror.

- If your tongue has a white coating, it could be a sign of infection, viral or bacterial. It can be resolved by sucking or drinking a vitamin C effervescent tablet. Most of the time, this is not a big problem.

- If your tongue appears red and white, your teeth get sensitive with warm or cold food -it could be a sign of acid reflux. Check the lower inside of your eyelids; if it is pale, you may need some iron supplement. Check with your doctor.

Difficulty in Breathing

- Use a Sinus Rinse to clean your nasal passage.

- Gurgle in your mouth and then suck on Takabb anti-cough pill from Thailand.

- Apply an electronic acupuncture pen on the seventh or fifth rib from the top down; it will stimulate the spleen to ease and open your breathing.

- Drink a glass of alkaline water with Fluimucil (acetylcysteine).

- Add a fluimucil (Acetylcysteine) effervescent tablet (sugar-free) into a cup of water to drink - it helps dry up the mucus before it spreads.

- Sleep on an Emtech machine (Bio cell charger). Lie chest down for easier breathing.

- An Emtech machine strengthens your bio-cell to aid muscle aches and recovery. Invented by an Australian-Singaporean research doctor, it releases oxygen, infrared red, long-wavelength, short-wavelength, and electromagnetic wave when activated.

Stomach Bloating

Too much sodium and potassium deficiency can cause bloating because potassium helps your body regulate excess fluid, reducing bloating. Too much sodium like salty foods causes water retention as cells hold on to excess water. Simply put, potassium and sodium need to be balanced to maintain the right equilibrium. Too much fluid retention can also cause you to gain water weight, known as edema - parts of your body become swollen with water.

The best way to avoid stomach bloating is to reduce your sodium and carbohydrate intake, drink more water to flush out excess sodium, and exercise regularly to sweat out excess water.

High Blood Pressure / Hypertension

The main causes of high blood pressure are:
- Overweight and obesity.

- Diet high in sodium and fat.

- Sedentary lifestyle.

- Stress.

- Excess alcohol and tobacco.

- Old age.

Should you have high blood pressure, lie down on the right side of your body. Take a few deep breaths and take your blood pressure. Your blood pressure should come down; take a rest breathing in this position. Learn to free your thoughts. Close your eyes and relax.

Lowering your high blood pressure naturally:

- Eat a low sodium diet.

- Limit your intake of alcohol to a maximum of 2 drinks for men and 1 drink for women.

- Exercise at least 30 minutes a day.

- Learn to manage your stress by learning to relax, e.g., walking outside or listening to relaxing music.

Headache

Take paracetamol, a common painkiller like Panadol or Tylenol. You can also use a cold pack and place it on your forehead for 15 minutes. If it is a tension headache, use a heating pad or hot compress and place it on the back of your head or neck.

Fever

Take Anarex, which also contains paracetamol to bring down fever, headache, and body aches. For a natural remedy, you can try squeezing juice from papaya leaves to drink.

Flu

According to doctors, the best way to prevent catching the flu is to get your flu vaccine. However, there are also other natural tips to prevent flu:

- Wash your hands regularly to avoid germs.

- Avoid touching your face as viruses can enter your body through your eyes, mouth, and nose.

- Consume more foods that contain phytochemicals, such as dark greens, red and yellow vegetables, and fruits.

- Cut down on alcohol and avoid smoking as this dries out your nasal passage making it susceptible for viruses to enter.

- Regularly exercising will get your heart pumping, thus increasing your body's natural virus-killing cells.

Diabetes

Drink soursop tea, nettle tea, green tea early in the morning, and before exercise. These teas are high in antioxidants and polyphenols; they are powerful compounds that play a role in preventing chronic diseases related to inflammation, such as diabetes, obesity, heart disease, and cancer. Drink these together with Alpha Lipoic acid for maximum effect (refer below).

Neem leaves powder is loaded with antioxidants and flavonoids. Anti-viral anti-inflammatory was found to control diabetic symptoms on non-insulin-dependent diabetics.

Cinnamon helps to improve blood sugar and cholesterol levels.
Fenugreek helps diabetic and boost libido.

Reduce carbohydrate intake. Avoid added sugar, trans-fat, and high-calorie foods in a diabetic diet. Having a healthy, nutritious diet can help to manage blood sugar levels.

Alpha-lipoic acid

Alpha-lipoic acid is an antioxidant that is more potent than vitamins C and E. It aids in preventing cell damage and restoring vitamin C and E levels in the body. It also helps to break down carbohydrates and turn them into energy for the body. Alpha-lipoic acid can help diabetes, as some studies have found that it helps improve insulin resistance.

Experiments have been done by injecting Alpha-lipoic acid into mice and removing the oxygen from the mice's container for a few hours. The container of mice without alpha-lipoic acid died. All the mice injected with alpha-lipoic acid still survive.

Research that includes large clinical trials supporting its role in treating neuropathy suggests it may help improve insulin sensitivity, lower blood sugar, cholesterol, decrease inflammation and oxidative stress.

<u>**Vitamin B12**</u>

Vitamin B12 deficiency can lead to anemia because your body does not have enough healthy red blood cells essential for carrying oxygen throughout your body. Side effects include:

- Tiredness

- Weakness

- Shortness of breath

- Light-headedness

- Poor balance

- Weight loss

- Depression

You can increase your vitamin B12 level with foods such as beef, liver, chicken, fish, shellfish, low-fat or fat-free milk, yogurt, cheese, eggs, and fortified breakfast cereals or vitamin B12 supplements.

<u>**Diet**</u>

Learn how diet can affect your health and make healthy choices. From my experience, diet is not about not eating, eating less, or skipping meals. You should learn about eating a little bit of everything that is important for your body. Do a medical checkup with a full blood test to balance your excess and deficiency.

My Tips on Diet:

1. Make changes to your diet. You are feeding the bacterial in your body that craved the food. They love sweet sugary food so try bitter food, e.g., kale, sprouts, bitter gourd, which is good for the liver, or drink low-fat milk.

2. Eat more protein, fruits, and vegetables. Most meat, fruits, and vegetables already have natural sugar in them.

3. Eat half a bowl of rice instead of your usual one or two bowls. Rice is sugar and carbohydrate.

4. Substitute your rice with more high fiber food, a spoonful of butter, and healthy fats, so that you will not go hungry faster. Do not snack. Avoid sugar and salt.

5. Avoid being a sweet tooth. Your body will fuel on the sugar first and not your fats. If your body cannot fuel on the sugar, it will have to fuel on your fats.

6. Stop eating cakes and ice-cream if you want to lose weight.

7. Drink more water to feed your hunger. Dehydration can cause you to believe you need to eat when you are actually thirsty.

8. Do more aerobic exercises that will increase your oxygen intake and heart rate, e.g., running, playing basketball, swimming, cycling, or stairs climbing.

9. Follow the adage of eating breakfast like a king, lunch like a prince, and dinner like a pauper. Don't go to bed right after a heavy dinner. You will put all the weight back on. If you can't sleep when you are hungry, take liquid food like Kefir, Fenugreek tea, and Chamomile tea.

10. Do not starve yourself. You do not need to suffer to achieve or attain anything. Merely find the correct way to do everything to maintain good health.

11. Avoid yo-yo dieting as you will feel weak, tired, lethargic, and fainting spells, etc.

12. Continue to learn, be disciplined, and committed, and you will improve and be in the best of health.

Kefir

Kefir is probiotic-rich fermented milk made from kefir grains. It works wonders for your gut by increasing the levels of healthy bacteria. It promotes digestion and helps the body absorb vitamins and minerals more effectively.

Fenugreek Tea

The seeds work wonders for digestion and promote the fat-burning process. They have anti-inflammatory properties and are rich in antioxidants. Drinking this tea before sleep can boost immunity and help you to detox.

Chamomile Tea

If you have difficulty sleeping, drinking this tea will help relax your nerves as it acts as a mild sedative; this tea also reduces glucose levels and promotes weight loss.

Magnesium

Magnesium, known as the master mineral, is responsible for more than 300 processes in the body. It helps regulate muscle and nerve functions and regulates blood sugar levels by reducing insulin. High magnesium reduces blood pressure and supplies protein, to the bones and DNA. Magnesium improves digestive health, relaxes intestinal muscles, attracts water to the intestine, soften stools preventing constipation, and eases anxiety and depression.

Magnesium deficiency can lead to calcium deficiency, poor heart health, muscle cramps, numbness, tingling sensations, tremors, nausea, high blood pressure, and respiratory illness. It is a nutrient that the body needs to stay healthy.

Squalene

One ingredient used in some COVID-19 vaccine candidates is squalene, natural oil made from the shark's liver. The shark is a mammal known for not having cancer even if cancer cells are injected into the shark. Squalene is now used to increase the effectiveness of the vaccine by creating a stronger immune response. It can soothe a variety of skin problems like eczema, psoriasis, dermatitis, and acne.

Coenzyme Q10 (CoQ10)

CoQ10, available in supplement form, is an antioxidant that your body produces naturally to aid in growth and maintenance, generating energy in your cells and protecting your cells from oxidative damage. Other benefits include improving heart function and keeping your skin young by promoting antioxidant protection.

Omega-3

Taking omega-3 supplements can help:

- Reduce risk factors for heart disease and cancer.

- Fight inflammation.

- Improve bone and joint health.

- Improve brain function.

- Improve eye health.

- Reduce fat in your liver.

Quercetin

Quercetin is a plant pigment known as flavonoids and found in many vegetables, fruits, and grains. It contains potent antioxidant properties and can be taken as a supplement, and its benefits include:

- Improves immunity.

- Prevents allergies.

- Fights inflammation.

- Improves general health.

Quercetin acts as an antioxidant, neutralizing free radicals that cause cellular and DNA damage. It is antibacterial and anti-inflammation. Take vitamin C with quercetin to lower high blood pressure.

Note: Clinical studies have shown that it could stop COVID-19 from infecting other cells in the body. The drawback is that it is not readily absorbed by the body and must be taken before the body is infected.

Honeysuckle

According to a study and clinical trial by researchers at Nanjing University, the herb honeysuckle has efficacy against SARS-CoV-2. The entire plant is used medically by the Chinese, Japanese, Thai, and Vietnamese. The dried flowers can also be used to treat arthritis, fever, headache, inflammation, increase urine flow, and prevent diarrhea. You can buy this herb and drink it as tea.

Watermelon

This fruit is rich in three blood pressure supporting nutrients, L-citrulline, lycopene, and potassium. It aids blood circulation.

L –citrulline produces nitric oxide, a gas that supports flexibility in arteries, relaxes blood vessels and helps lower blood pressure.

Lycopene – Food that is red or pink in color is rich in lycopene, an antioxidant that positively affects high blood pressure.

<u>**White Color Foods**</u>

The Chinese believe that food that is white in color nourishes the lungs, promotes urination, and reduces heatiness. Porridge, barley, oats, white fungus is taken if one falls sick with a cough, flu, and fever. Food white in color helps with improving appetite and recovery.

<u>**Nourishing Tea**</u>

Boil red dates, longans, white fungus, ginkgo seeds, brown sugar together to make a tea and drink to warm up the body before winter. This ancient recipe also helps strengthen the immune system.

<u>**Potential Treatments from Around the World:**</u>

- According to a Japanese study, amino-acids cysteine and theanine could have efficacy against SARS-CoV-2.

- German Researchers confirm that extracts of the plant Artemisia Annua are active against SARS-CoV-2.

- Russian study indicates Glutathione deficiency affects COVID-19 susceptibility, supplement N-AcetylCysteine (NAC) helps.

- Researchers at Yale School of Medicine advocates a ketogenic diet, which is low in carbohydrate and high in fat, could have possible benefits for elderly COVID-19 patients.

- Chinese physicians smoke herbs through dragon fire moxibustion acupuncture of the meridian points into your spinal bones to treat your symptoms.

- Catalase is an antioxidant enzyme found in liver, erythrocytes, and alveolar epithelial cells to protect the body from oxidative cell damage. It is also available as a low-cost supplement. Researchers at the School of Medicine at the University of California found that this enzyme offers an effective therapeutic solution for the treatment of hyper-inflammation in SARS-CoV-2 patients.

The difference in treatments between the eastern and western medicine is the western medicine weakens the body as the medicine takes effect to help the body recover, in contrast with eastern medicine that believes in strengthening the body so the immune system can take over the healing role. Ask yourself why the West, during this pandemic, has no medicine to deal with this crisis while China can treat 1.4 billion people with TCM to lessen the virus's effect before turning to the research of vaccine?

You can be taught how to breathe and exercise, you can consult your doctor, but these are not enough. You have to exercise to keep yourself healthy. Don't only read, really exercise and make time to get some sunlight, if not only for 15 minutes three times a day.

We need to maintain good blood circulation, deep breathing, exercises, take magnesium, potassium, and many other ways to detox. The amount of toxic we have build-up over the years can make our health very poor.

Chapter 5 - Useful Things to Keep at Home

"When diet is wrong, medicine is no use. When diet is correct, medicine is of no need." -Ayurvedic proverb

Create a checklist to cater to your needs. Here are my suggestions:

1) Personal medication - consult your doctor.

2) Anarex - relieves body aches and headache.

3) Multi-vitamins - especially important ones like Vitamin D, B12, and magnesium.

4) Lycopene - promotes healthy eyesight and high blood pressure.

5) Psyllium - aids digestion by soaking up water in your gut and making your bowel movement regular. It improves heart health by managing cholesterol levels.

6) Caraway essential oil - helps with bloating, reduces inflammation, and supports immune health.

7) Cat's claw - helps ease symptoms of rheumatoid arthritis.

8) Fluimucil (acetylcysteine) effervescent tablets - helps clear mucus and phlegm.

9) Eno fruit salt - relieve for indigestion, stomach upset, and heatiness.

10) Kefentech plaster - relieve for muscle aches, stiffness, strains, and joint pain.

11) Gaviscon - relieves heartburn and indigestion from overeating.

12) CoQ10 - provides energy to cells.

13) Uniflu - treats cold and flu symptoms.

14) Qing Fei Pai Du Tang - clearing of lungs and body detox.

15) Licorice tea - soothes an upset stomach, heartburn, and acid reflux.

16) Electronic acupuncture pen - used to target your 7th left rib from below lowest is the twelfth rib. It will vibrate your spleen and help your lungs to breathe.

17) Toothache tea - relieves toothache, inflammation, and sore throat as effectively as neuflo tablets.

18) Watermelon Frost Powder spray - relieves inflammation and throat pain.

19) Cardiprin tablets - lowers the risk of stroke and heart attack in people with blood vessel disorders. Each tablet contains 100mg of aspirin and 45mg glycine and can be taken by dissolving it on the tongue or with a glass of water.

Note: Please seek your doctor's advice before taking any medicine.

Chapter 6 - Personal Hygiene

"Hygiene is two-thirds of health." -Lebanese proverb

Some of us may think that we practice personal hygiene fairly well. The truth is what you are currently doing might not be enough because we are not living in normal conditions due to the COVID-19 pandemic.

When you are at home, do you let your guard down? Do you head for the shower the minute you reach home? My advice is to not interact with your family members until you have bathed. You do not want to risk infecting them with any germs that might be residing on your clothes and followed you home.

Consider chlorine steam or ozone air used together with the air conditioner in your house or car to sterilize your surrounding and clothing.

Note: When you UV your room, you should not be in the room. The UV light and ozone air will tighten your skin and is harmful to your skin when overexposed. The ozone air will damage some of your cells as well as viruses near your opening. You will breathe in deeply, hoping to kill, weaken, or damage more viruses near the opening of your nose and mouth. You might look slightly younger, though, as the ozone tightens the skin and removes wrinkles for a brief moment.

Some patients are still tested positive months after their quarantine because they keep breathing in the virus in their surroundings. Sterilize the whole room if required. Minimize the amount of virus infecting your body by washing and cleaning up as often as you can. Detox frequently to cleanse your internal body. I used clear lungs herbal body detox from the Chinese medical hall.

Every night I close my room and sterilize it with a UV light that also produces ozone air before sleeping. At the same time, I open the main door to allow more oxygen to enter through my locked grille gates.

Use a sinus rinsing kit, Audisol for clearing blocked ears, nasal sprays for a blocked nose (you can only spray a maximum of 4 days a week), and Snorel spray for breathing easy while you sleep. I use these to take in more oxygen into my body while resting.

Clean your house every day with Dettol before you rest. I like to add peach shampoo to the Dettol for a better fragrance. Singapore National Environment Agency approved only 3 types of antiseptic shampoo from Dettol. You can check the Dettol website for more information.

I use Betadine tea tree and aloe vera body wash, which claims to kill 99.99% germs with its gentle formula enriched with vitamin E. I use baby wipes to clean myself when I am uncomfortable with certain car rides. I can shower as many as six times a day just to ensure I keep my family and myself as safe as possible. Whatever you do, be mindful and always be safe.

Vitamin	Benefits	Good Food Sources
Vitamin A *(Retinol, Retinal, and Retinoic Acid)*	Essential for vision Lowers risk of prostate cancer Keeps tissue and skin healthy Helps in bone growth Lowers risk of lung cancer Carotenoids act as antioxidants Foods rich in carotenoids, lutein, and zeaxanthin may protect against cataracts	Sources of Retinoid : Beef Liver Eggs Prawns Fish Fortified Milk Cheddar and Swiss Cheese Sources of Beta Carotene : Sweet Potatoes Carrots Pumpkin Squash Spinach Mangoes Turnip Greens
Vitamin B_1 *(Thiamin)*	Helps convert food into energy Needed for healthy skin, hair, muscles, and brain	Pork Chops Ham Soymilk Watermelons Acorn Squash

Vitamin B$_2$ (Riboflavin)	Helps convert food into energy Needed for healthy skin, hair, blood, and brain	Milk Yogurt Cheese Whole and Enriched Grains Cereals Liver
Vitamin B$_3$ (Niacin)	Helps convert food into energy Needed for healthy skin, blood cells, nervous system, and brain	Meat Poultry Fish Fortified and Whole Grains Mushrooms Potatoes Peanut Butter
Vitamin B$_5$ (Pantothenic Acid)	Helps convert food into energy Helps make lipids, neurotransmitters, steroid hormones, and hemoglobin	Chicken Whole Grains Broccoli Mushrooms Avocados Tomato Products
Vitamin B$_6$ (Pyridoxal, Pyridoxine, Pyridoxamine)	Aids in lowering homocysteine levels and may reduce the risk of heart diseases Helps convert tryptophan to niacin and serotonin (a	Meat Fish Poultry

	neurotransmitter that plays key roles in sleep, appetite, and moods) Helps make red blood cells Influences cognitive abilities and immune function	Legumes Tofu and Other Soy Products Potatoes Non-Citrus Fruits
Vitamin B$_{12}$ *(Cobalamin)*	Aids in lowering homocysteine levels and may reduce the risk of heart diseases Assists in making new cells and breaking down some fatty acids and amino acids Protects nerve cells and encourages their normal growth Helps make red blood cells	Meat Fish Poultry Milk Cheese Eggs Fortified Cereals Fortified Soymilk
Vitamin B$_7$ *(Biotin)*	Helps convert food into energy and synthesize glucose Helps make and break down some fatty acids Needed for healthy bones and hair	Whole Grains Organ Meats Egg Yolks Soybeans Fish
Vitamin C *(Ascorbic Acid)*	May lower risk of some cancers Long term use of supplemental Vitamin C may protect against cataracts Helps make collagen (a connective tissue that knits together wounds and supports blood vessel walls) Helps make neurotransmitters, serotonin and norepinephrine	Fruit and Fruit Juices (especially citrus) Potatoes Broccoli Bell peppers Spinach

	Acts as an antioxidant, neutralize unstable molecules that can damage cells Bolsters the immune system	Strawberries Tomatoes Brussels Sprouts
Choline	Helps make and release the neurotransmitter acetylcholine, which aids in many nerve and brain activities Plays a role in metabolism and transporting fats	Milk Eggs Liver Peanuts
Vitamin D *(Calciferous)*	Helps maintain normal blood levels of calcium and phosphorus that strengthens bones Helps form teeth and bones Supplements can reduce the number of non-spinal fractures	Fortified Milk or Margarine Fortified Cereals Fatty Fish
Vitamin E *(Alpha-Tocopherol)*	Acts as an antioxidant, neutralize unstable molecules that can damage cells Protects Vitamin A and certain lipids from damage Diets rich in Vitamin E may help prevent Alzheimer's Disease Supplements may protect against prostate cancer	Vegetable Oils Salad Dressings Wheat Germ Leafy Green Vegetables Whole Grains Nuts
Folic Acid	Vital for new cell creation Helps prevent brain and spine birth defects when taken early in	Fortified Grains and Cereals Asparagus

	pregnancy Can lower levels of homocysteine and may reduce the risk of heart disease May reduce the risk of colon cancer Offsets risk of breast cancer among women who consume alcohol	Okra Spinach Turnip Greens Legumes Orange Juice Tomato Juice
Vitamin K *(Phylloquinone, menadione)*	Activates proteins and calcium essential to blood clotting May help prevents hip fractures	Cabbage Liver Eggs Milk Spinach Broccoli Sprouts Kale Collards

Conclusion

I hope that everyone who reads this book will find information to improve your health and strengthen your body.

As a taxi driver, I have to sit still in the car for long hours every day. I have to focus on taking deep breaths so that the oxygen can reach my fingers and toes. I also exercise by opening and closing my fingers and toes, which is another way to improve blood circulation and not get the economy class syndrome.

If you can afford it, get a personal trainer or a yoga instructor to help you work out. Most importantly, you must have discipline and commitment to your health and wellbeing.

I am poor, I work very hard, I have my problems, but I am not giving up. This is my first book, and I sincerely hope I can help as many people as possible with my personal knowledge and experience.

Remember, when the going gets tough, the tough get going.

Live your life. Don't give up.

Yours sincerely,
ERNIE ONG

References

https://www.healthline.com/nutrition/13-habits-linked-to-a-long-life#:~:text=Longevity%20may%20seem%20beyond%20your,path%20to%20a%20long%20life.

https://www.ncbi.nlm.nih.gov/pmc/articles/PMC2287209/

https://en.wikipedia.org/wiki/Huangdi_Neijing

https://www.ncbi.nlm.nih.gov/pmc/articles/PMC5689451/

https://www.healthline.com/nutrition/vitamin-d-from-sun#overview

https://my.clevelandclinic.org/health/articles/15050-vitamin-d--vitamin-d-deficiency

https://www.health.com/nutrition/vitamins-supplements/vitamin-d-benefits

https://www.bbc.com/news/health-15151930#:~:text=Most%20people%20get%20enough%20vitamin,oily%20fish%20and%20dairy%20products.

https://www.bhachc.org/much-sunlight-enough/

https://www.terrapinadventures.com/blog/exercise-fresh-air-health/#:~:text=Fresh%20air%20is%20good%20for,leading%20to%20a%20healthier%20you.

http://liwli.com/surprising-health-benefits-of-fresh-air/

https://www.mayoclinichealthsystem.org/hometown-health/speaking-of-health/water-essential-to-your-body#:~:text=Here%20are%20just%20a%20few%20important%20ways%20water%20works%20in%20your%20body%3A&text=Protects%20body%20organs%20and%20tissues,by%20flushing%20out%20waste%20products

https://www.healthline.com/health/food-nutrition/why-is-water-important#nutrients

https://www.healthline.com/health-news/2-hours-dehydration-can-affect-body-and-brain#What-did-they-find?-

https://www.usgs.gov/special-topic/water-science-school/science/water-you-water-and-human-body?qt-science_center_objects=0#qt-science_center_objects

https://www.cdc.gov/media/releases/2016/p0215-enough-sleep.html

https://www.medicalnewstoday.com/articles/best-time-to-sleep-and-wake-up#going-to-sleep

https://www.who.int/teams/health-promotion/physical-activity/physical-activity-and-adults

https://www.health.harvard.edu/newsletter_article/how-much-exercise-do-you-need

https://www.healthline.com/health/fitness/alcohol-before-workout-safe#:~:text=Alcohol%20is%20a%20depressant%2C%20meaning,to%20be%20less%20than%20optimal.

https://www.health.harvard.edu/cold-and-flu/can-vitamin-c-prevent-a-cold#:~:text=The%20impact%20on%20colds&text=More%20encouraging%3A%20taking%20at%20least,one%20less%20day%20of%20illness.

https://en.wikipedia.org/wiki/List_of_citrus_fruits

https://www.webmd.com/diet/features/the-benefits-of-vitamin-c#1

https://betteryou.com/health-hub/magnesium-vitamin-d-benefits-dosages-types-supplements/

https://en.wikipedia.org/wiki/COVID-19_pandemic

https://en.wikipedia.org/wiki/2002%E2%80%932004_SARS_outbreak

https://www.ncbi.nlm.nih.gov/pmc/articles/PMC7462404/

https://www.ncbi.nlm.nih.gov/pmc/articles/PMC7293495/

https://www.nationalgeographic.com/science/2020/06/could-flushing-public-toilet-plume-spread-coronavirus-cvd/

https://www.epa.gov/coronavirus/indoor-air-homes-and-coronavirus-covid-19

https://www.thailandmedical.news/news/breaking-coronavirus-news-chinese-study-shows-that-pillows-made-from-microfibers-can-be-reservoirs-for-sars-cov-2-coronavirus

https://time.com/5899294/reinfection-coronavirus/

https://www.health.harvard.edu/staying-healthy/how-to-boost-your-immune-system

https://www.resilience.org/stories/2020-04-23/fraying-food-system-may-be-our-next-crisis/

https://difflam.sg/product/difflam-sore-throat-lozenges/

https://todayspractitioner.com/traditional-chinese-medicine-tcm/qing-fei-pai-du-tang-herbal-formula-for-integrative-covid-19-therapies-in-china/#.X41N1dAzaUk

https://www.healthline.com/nutrition/how-to-detox-your-body#TOC_TITLE_HDR_6

https://www.lifehack.org/articles/lifestyle/17-toxic-fruits-and-vegetables-you-may-eating-every-day.html

https://www.healthline.com/health/carotenoids

https://www.aarp.org/health/drugs-supplements/info-08-2010/toxic-drugs-when-medicine-makes-you-sick.html

https://www.verywellmind.com/toxicity-meaning-and-signs-and-symptoms-1067226

https://www.webmd.com/vitamins-and-supplements/activated-charcoal-uses-risks#1

https://www.healthline.com/nutrition/activated-charcoal#:~:text=Activated%20charcoal%20is%20a%20fine,it%20at%20very%20high%20temperatures.

https://www.avogel.co.uk/food/can-potassium-help-with-bloating/

https://www.medicalnewstoday.com/articles/320603

https://www.medicalnewstoday.com/articles/320603#ways-to-lose-water-weight

https://familydoctor.org/condition/high-blood-pressure/

https://www.goodrx.com/blog/fastest-way-to-lower-blood-pressure-safely/

https://www.webmd.com/migraines-headaches/5-ways-to-get-rid-of-headache

https://www.drugs.com/international/anarex.html

https://www.webmd.com/cold-and-flu/11-tips-prevent-cold-flu#1

https://www.berkeley.edu/news/media/releases/96legacy/releases.96/1
4316.html#:~:text=2%2F21%2F96-
,A%20relatively%20unknown%20antioxidant%2C%20alpha%2Dlipoic%
20acid%2C%20may%20be,than%20vitamins%20C%20and%20E

https://www.webmd.com/vitamins/ai/ingredientmono-767/alpha-lipoic-
acid

https://www.webmd.com/diabetes/supplement-guide-alpha-lipoic-
acid#:~:text=We%20have%20strong%20evidence%20that,by%20diab
etes%20or%20cancer%20treatment.

https://www.webmd.com/a-to-z-guides/vitamin-b12-deficiency-
anemia#1

https://medium.com/@BSXTechnologies/how-drinking-more-water-
5b5b94a610cb#:~:text=Thirst%20occurs%20when%20your%20body,y
ou%20really%20need%20liquid%20intake.

https://en.wikipedia.org/wiki/Kefir

https://www.healthline.com/nutrition/9-health-benefits-of-
kefir#TOC_TITLE_HDR_3

https://www.deccanherald.com/living/magnesium-master-mineral-
720212.html

https://news.sky.com/story/coronavirus-half-a-million-sharks-could-be-
killed-for-vaccine-experts-warn-12083167

https://www.healthline.com/nutrition/coenzyme-q10

https://www.mayoclinic.org/drugs-supplements-coenzyme-q10/art-
20362602

https://www.healthline.com/nutrition/17-health-benefits-of-omega-
3#TOC_TITLE_HDR_2

https://www.medpagetoday.com/infectiousdisease/covid19/87373

https://www.thailandmedical.news/news/breaking-news-covid-19-herbs-
researchers-confirms-that-in-studies-and-clinical-trials-the-herb-
honeysuckle-has-efficacy-against-sars-cov-2

https://www.thailandmedical.news/news/breaking-news-artemisia-
annua-german-researchers-confirm-that-extracts-of-the-plant-
artemisia-annua-are-active-against-sars-cov-2-coronavirus

https://www.thailandmedical.news/news/ketogenic-diet-and-covid-19-yale-led-study-advocates-keto-diet-for-elderly-covid-19-patients-due-to-possible-benefits-and-better-clinical-outcomes#:~:text=Ketogenic%20Diet%20And%20COVID%2D19%3A%20Researchers%20in%20a%20new%20study,patients%20and%20even%20those%20not

http://www.sci-news.com/medicine/catalase-covid-19-08921.html

https://www.healthline.com/health/psyllium-health-benefits

https://www.thegoldenconcepts.com/products/kefentech-air-plaster

https://www.gaviscon.com.sg/

https://www.healthline.com/nutrition/licorice-root#uses

https://www.amcal.com.au/cardiprin-tablets-100mg-90-tablets-p-9300631015185

https://www.mims.com/malaysia/drug/info/cardiprin%20100?type=full#:~:text=Aspirin%20100%20mg%2C%20glycine%2045%20mg.&text=Each%20tablet%20contains%20aspirin%20100,(aminoacetic%20acid)%2045%20mg.
https://www.healthline.com/health-news/change-clothes-to-get-rid-of-germs

www.ingramcontent.com/pod-product-compliance
Lightning Source LLC
Chambersburg PA
CBHW061531250726

48657CB00005B/2174